MENTAL HEALTH COOKBOOK FOR SENIORS

The Complete and Optimal Mental Wellness Guide with Healthy Recipes to Prevent Alzheimers, Cognitive Decline and Dementia.

EPIPHANY HUB PRINTS

MENTAL HEALTH COOKBOOK FOR SENIORS

COPYRIGHT © [2023] BY [EPIPHANY HUB PRINTS]

TABLE OF CONTENTS

INTRODUCTION

There is a strong relationship between our mental health and the foods we eat when it comes to nutrition and wellbeing. This link becomes even more important as we age gracefully, which emphasizes the need of a balanced diet catered to the special requirements of older citizens. Welcome to the "Mental Health Cookbook for Seniors"—a gastronomic adventure that feeds the mind and body alike.

As a nutritionist, I have had the honor of seeing firsthand how food can significantly improve the lives of numerous elderly people. It is well known that diet and physical health are related, but in this cookbook, we aim to explore the complex relationship between diet and mental health. We set out on this journey not only as guardians of our physical bodies but also as stewards of our mental health.

The golden years should be a time of happiness, contentment, and abundant experiences, but they can also bring special difficulties that might be detrimental to one's mental health. Feelings of loneliness and sadness can be exacerbated by physical illnesses, the aging process, loneliness, and the loss of loved ones.

But the foundation of our strategy is empowerment: we think that seniors can take charge of their mental health and fully enjoy life if they are equipped with the correct information and resources.

This cookbook is a comprehensive guide that combines the art of culinary handicraft with the science of nutrition, not just a list of recipes. These pages will provide the techniques for choosing substances that support emotional equilibrium, lower stress levels, and improve cognitive performance.

We'll look at the function of antioxidants, vital nutrients, and the amazing potential of culinary herbs to improve mental wellness. You will learn about the delights of meal planning, mindful eating, and enjoying hearty meals with those you care about.

You will discover a veritable gold mine of delectable and nutritious dishes in the pages that follow, many of which support the ideas of helping seniors maintain their mental health. You will be actively creating a life that is healthier, happier, and more rewarding with every bite.

Together, let's embark on this culinary journey and allow the flavors and smells of carefully prepared dishes to inspire a fresh enthusiasm for life. Here's to a gastronomic and mental wellness adventure with the "Mental Health Cookbook for Seniors."

THANK YOU VERY MUCH FOR TAKING YOUR TIME TO READ THIS BOOK. I FOUND JOY SHARING MY THOUGHTS WITH YOU. HAVING ENJOYED "**MENTAL HEALTH COOKBOOK FOR SENIORS**", I WOULD DROP OUR EMAIL AS A MEANS OF REACHING OUT.

MEANWHILE I SENT OUT READING LIST OF MY FAVORITE BOOKS FROM MYSELF AND OTHER AUTHORS ON A WIDE RANGE OF SUBJECTS.

epiphanyhubprints@gmail.com

I ALWAYS HAVE A GIFT FOR EVERYONE THAT REACHED OUT!

"Cooking with Love, Serving with Care."

CHAPTER 1:

MENTAL HEALTH AND NUTRITION

Our "Mental Health Cookbook for Seniors" begins with a chapter that defines the basic concepts of the complex interrelationship between the mind and body. We explore the deep relationships that exist between physical and mental health in this area.

Understanding the Mind-Body Connection

Here, we examine the reciprocal effects of our ideas, feelings, and actions on our physical well-being. We stress how important it is to understand that our physical and nutritional habits have a significant impact on our mental health. Seniors need to understand this since it is the foundation of the holistic approach that we promote in the cookbook.

The Importance of Nutrition in Senior Mental Health

In this section, we discuss the special dietary requirements of the elderly and the critical role that good nutrition plays in preserving and improving mental health as we age. We explore the science underlying the ways in which nutrition and nutrients might affect mental health, emotional stability, and general quality of life.

Goals and Structure of the Cookbook

We lay out the goals and organization of the cookbook to set the scene for the remainder of the book. Our main objective is to provide seniors with the information and resources they need to make wise dietary decisions, which will improve their mental health results. We go over how the following chapters are structured to give seniors, caregivers, and medical professionals a clear road map.

The layout of the cookbook is intended to be user-friendly, featuring simple-to-follow recipes, meal plans, and helpful advice. The ultimate goal is to support mental health by utilizing the power of mindful eating, establishing a harmonic and balanced relationship between the body and mind so that seniors can lead full and satisfying lives.

Beginning with a firm understanding of the relationship between mind and body, the role that nutrition plays in senior mental health, and the objectives and format of the cookbook, readers are prepared to use the recipes and advice found in the following chapters to set out on a path toward better mental health and general well-being.

"NOURISH THE MIND, FEED THE SOUL."

CHAPTER 2:

SENIORS' UNIQUE NUTRITIONAL NEEDS

Nutritional Requirements for Aging Adults

Understanding these shifting requirements is essential for preserving both physical and mental health as people age and their nutritional requirements change. These needs must be addressed in a senior mental health cookbook in order to promote cognitive well-being. Important things to think about are:

Reduced Metabolism: A slowed metabolism is a common consequence of aging. While the number of calories needed by seniors may decrease, the quality of those calories becomes even more important for mental well-being.

Protein for Brain Health: Eating a diet high in protein is essential for protecting and rebuilding brain tissue. To promote cognitive function, place an emphasis on lean protein sources including fish, chicken, legumes, and low-fat dairy.

Fiber and the Gut-Brain Connection: Eating a diet rich in fiber helps improve gut health, which in turn has a significant impact on mental health. Encourage the consumption of fruits, vegetables, and whole grains to support a balanced gut microbiome.

Hydration: It's critical to provide advice on sustaining an appropriate fluid intake because dehydration can aggravate cognitive problems.

Common Nutritional Deficiencies in Seniors

To assist seniors in avoiding these problems and maintaining their mental health, it is imperative to draw attention to the prevalent dietary inadequacies that they experience. These shortcomings may consist of:

Vitamin D: Seniors are more likely to become deficient in this nutrient due to decreased sun exposure and decreased ability to synthesis it. For optimal brain function, vitamin D levels must be maintained by food, or supplements may be required.

Vitamin B12: B12 is necessary for cognitive function and its absorption may be hampered by an age-related decrease in stomach acid. Encourage B12 sources such as lean meats and fortified cereals.

Calcium: Inadequate calcium intake affects mental health indirectly and is essential for strong bones in many elderly people. Promote the eating of leafy greens, dairy products, and fortified plant-based milk.

Omega-3 Fatty Acids: Seniors frequently don't get enough omega-3 fatty acids in their diet, despite the fact that they are crucial for brain function. Encourage the consumption of walnuts, flaxseeds, and fatty fish as sources of these healthy fats.

Tailoring Your Diet to Mental Well-being:

Seniors can adopt certain food choices that have a favorable impact on their well-being to preserve and improve their mental health. You can give them dietary advice based on your mental health cookbook:

Anti-Inflammatory Foods: To help lower the risk of cognitive decline, emphasize foods that have anti-inflammatory qualities, such as berries, turmeric, and leafy greens.

Mediterranean Diet: Research has linked enhanced cognitive function to a diet high in fruits, vegetables, whole grains, and olive oil. Provide meal ideas and dishes that follow this nutritional trend.

Balanced Macronutrients: To maintain stable blood sugar levels and mood control, promote a balance of healthy fats, proteins, and carbohydrates.

Mindful Eating: Encourage elders to adopt mindful eating habits to help them enjoy their food more and feel more satisfied after eating.

"A Healthy Plate, A Happy State."

CHAPTER 3:

BRAIN-BOOSTING NUTRIENTS

Particularly for older adults, omega-3 fatty acids are vital nutrients that are critical for preserving and enhancing cognitive function. You can stress in your senior mental health cookbook the value of include foods high in omega-3 fatty acids, such walnuts, flaxseeds, and fatty fish (salmon, mackerel, and sardines).

Reduced cognitive decline, improved memory and cognitive function, and a decreased risk of age-related mental health conditions including dementia and Alzheimer's disease have all been associated with omega-3 fatty acids.

Incorporate meal ideas that highlight these foods high in omega-3s, such as a salad with avocado and salmon or a fish dish with a walnut crust. Tell your readers how adding these nutrients to their diet on a regular basis can improve mental clarity and general wellbeing.

Brain Health and Antioxidants:

Strong substances called antioxidants guard the brain against oxidative stress and inflammation, two things that can impede cognitive function. An antioxidant-rich diet, which includes foods like berries, dark leafy greens, and vibrant veggies, is beneficial for seniors. Emphasize in your cookbook the value of these colorful foods and how they support brain health.

Provide recipes that use foods high in antioxidants, like a salad of spinach and kale with an assortment of vibrant veggies or a smoothie with mixed berries. Highlight the ways in which these antioxidants can enhance general mental health and lower the risk of age-related cognitive decline.

Minerals and Vitamins for Mood and Memory

Seniors' mental health depends on certain vitamins and minerals for mood regulation and memory maintenance. Your cookbook should have information on the significance of certain nutrients, such as magnesium, vitamin D, and the vitamin B complex. These nutrients have a favorable effect on mood and mental clarity.

Provide recipes that use foods rich in these vital minerals and vitamins. To increase vitamin D intake, for instance, include a segment of recipes that highlight foods high in folate, a B vitamin, such as leafy greens and legumes, or dishes that include fatty fish and fortified dairy products. Seniors can make educated dietary decisions that improve their mental health by learning how these nutrients enhance mood, memory, and general mental health.

Including these subjects in your senior mental health cookbook will not only turn it into a useful tool but also give seniors the confidence to use their diet to take control of their mental health.

With this knowledge, they will be able to make wise decisions and savor delectable, brain-boosting meals that support their general mental health, mood regulation, and cognitive performance.

"From Garden to Gratitude: Cultivating Mental Wellness."

CHAPTER 4:

MEAL PLANNING FOR A HEALTHY MIND

Crafting a Well-Balanced Diet

For seniors in particular, sustaining optimal mental health requires a well-balanced diet. Choosing a variety of nutrient-rich foods that include important vitamins, minerals, and other critical components is part of creating a diet that promotes mental well-being. This is how you do it:

Various Food Groups: Try to include a variety of food groups, such as whole grains, fruits, vegetables, lean meats, and healthy fats. Every dietary type has special advantages for the health of the brain and body.

Dish of Color: Arrange a variety of vibrant fruits and vegetables on your dish. As different hues correspond to different nutrients, eating a rainbow of vegetables can be very good for your mental well-being.

Lean Protein Sources: These include tofu, fish, poultry, and lentils. These supply the amino acids required for the synthesis of neurotransmitters, which are essential for controlling mood.

Whole Grains: Choose whole wheat bread, brown rice, and quinoa among other whole grains. These complex carbs help to normalize blood sugar levels and improve mental clarity by releasing energy gradually.

Healthy Fats: Include foods high in unsaturated fats, like almonds, avocados, and olive oil. These fats can help with better cognitive function and are vital for the health of the brain.

Calorie Requirements and Portion Control

Maintaining a healthy body weight and promoting mental wellness both depend on portion control. Seniors who consume too many calories should be careful because doing so can result in weight gain and other mental health problems. How to control calorie needs and portion sizes is as follows:

Recognize Your BMR (Basal Metabolic Rate): To find out how many calories you need each day based on your age, gender, weight, and level of activity, calculate your BMR. This will assist you in determining your baseline caloric consumption.

Balanced Meals: Make sure to consume a daily allowance of calories in small meals and snacks. To maintain steady energy levels throughout the day, make sure each meal consists of a combination of macronutrients (fats, proteins, and carbohydrates).

Eating with awareness: Pay attention to your body's signals of hunger and fullness. A more attentive connection with food can be fostered and overeating can be avoided.

Portion Size Awareness: To assist in regulating portion sizes, use smaller plates and cutlery. Your brain may be tricked into thinking that consuming less food will satisfy you.

Tips for Managing Special Dietary Requirements

Due to a variety of medical issues, seniors may have specific dietary requirements or limits. It's critical to balance these demands with the advancement of mental wellness. The following advice can help you cater to specific dietary needs:

Speak with a Healthcare Professional: Speak with a certified dietitian or healthcare practitioner if you have any special dietary needs or medical issues. They can assist you in developing a customized diet plan that satisfies your needs and promotes mental wellness.

Allergies and Intolerances: Recognize and steer clear of foods that cause an intolerance or allergy. To guarantee that you can still eat a range of meals safely, there are many of substitute ingredients available.

Medication Interactions: Keep in mind that there may be a conflict between some meals and prescription drugs. Dietary changes may be necessary for certain drugs to stay effective.

Support from Caregivers: If your health prevents you from cooking, ask your caregivers for help or consider food delivery services that might meet your dietary requirements.

These standards ensure that the recipes and dietary recommendations in a senior mental health cookbook meet personal tastes, dietary needs, and constraints while also supporting physical and mental well-being.

CHAPTER 5:

RECIPES FOR COGNITIVE HEALTH

For seniors, maintaining good cognitive function is critical, and nutrition is a key factor in attaining this. This chapter explores the two most important meals of the day, breakfast and lunch, and provides you with recipes that are specifically crafted to improve mental clarity, focus, and brain health in general.

Breakfast: Intelligence-Spurring Starters

1. Blueberry and Walnut Overnight Oats: This recipe is a nutritional powerhouse that will enhance your brain function. Antioxidants found in blueberries shield brain cells, and omega-3 fatty acids found in walnuts are beneficial to cognition. Additionally, oats provide a continuous energy release that helps you stay focused throughout the morning.

2. Spinach and Feta Omelette: Packed with spinach, which is high in folate, a nutrient crucial for brain function, this

omelette is tasty and healthful. Feta cheese offers additional protein and a creamy touch.

3. Green Tea and Almond Smoothie: Packed with vitamin E and good fats that promote memory and general cognitive function, almonds go well with green tea, which is recognized for its ability to improve cognition.

Lunch: Energizing Midday Meals

1. Salmon and Quinoa Salad: This recipe pairs omega-3-rich salmon, which is good for the brain, with quinoa, a high-protein grain that gives you prolonged energy and helps you stay focused throughout the afternoon.

2. Lentil and Vegetable Soup: A filling soup made with a variety of veggies and lentils. While the vegetables provide a range of vital nutrients for preserving cognitive function, lentils are a great source of folate.

3. Avocado and Turkey Wrap: Avocados are high in heart-healthy lipids that are good for the brain. Serve it with lean turkey, whole-grain wraps, and an assortment of vegetables for a filling and cognitively stimulating meal.

4. Berry and Kale Power Salad: A colorful salad with kale, berries, and a dash of almonds. Antioxidants are found in berries, and vitamin K is abundant in kale, which supports mental clarity and brain health.

Dinner: Nourishing the Mind and Body

Dinner is frequently seen as the focal point of family get-togethers and has a big impact on senior mental health. We examine the relationship between supper and emotional health in this chapter. We provide meal plans and dishes that encourage unwinding, lower stress levels, and improve mental health in general, making supper an occasion to look forward to.

Dinner Plates That Are Well-Balanced: Discover how to put together dinner plates that are well-balanced and include a range of nutrients that are vital for mental wellness. We stress the value of including plenty of colorful veggies, healthy grains, and lean proteins.

Practices of Mindful Eating: This section delves into the idea of mindful eating, urging seniors to relish their food, appreciate its flavors, and practice relaxing techniques while they eat.

"Recipes for Resilience: Cooking Through Life's Seasons."

CHAPTER 6:

NUTRITIONAL STRATEGIES FOR MANAGING STRESS AND ANXIETY

How Nutrition Impacts Stress Levels

Stress levels are greatly influenced by nutrition, which is particularly important for seniors who want to keep their mental health. Our diets have the power to either reduce or increase stress. As follows:

Blood Sugar Regulation: Eating a diet high in fiber, lean proteins, and complex carbs helps to keep blood sugar levels stable. Stress levels can rise and mood swings can result from blood sugar fluctuations. For steady blood sugar levels, seniors should prioritize veggies, healthy grains, and lean meats.

Micronutrients: The synthesis of neurotransmitters that control mood depends on a number of vitamins and minerals, including magnesium and B-vitamins. Stress and anxiety may worsen if there is a nutrient deficit. Consuming items that supply these, such as whole grains, nuts, and leafy greens

Omega-3 Fatty Acids: Rich sources of anti-inflammatory characteristics, omega-3 fatty acids can help lower stress levels. They can be found in walnuts and fatty seafood like salmon. These beneficial fats can help to soothe the mind and boost brain function.

Alcohol and Caffeine: Seniors should use caution while consuming either of these substances. Although a cup of coffee could provide a little energy boost, consuming too much of it might cause anxiety and restlessness. In a similar vein, excessive alcohol consumption can worsen stress and interfere with sleep cycles.

Foods that Help You Chill

There are meals that are proven to provide calming and relaxing effects. For seniors, including these in your diet may help with better mental health:

Herbal Teas: Due to their inherent calming properties, chamomile, lavender, and lemon balm teas can aid in stress relief and relaxation.

Dark Chocolate: When consumed in moderation, dark chocolate with a high cocoa content might cause endorphins to be released, which will make you feel happy and relaxed.

Nuts: Packed with magnesium, almonds and walnuts may help soothe the nervous system.

Fruits: Tryptophan and potassium, which are found in bananas, can help calm the body and regulate mood. Fruits' inherent sugars can give off a mild energy boost.

Whole Grains: Complex carbohydrates included in whole grains, such as quinoa and oats, help to produce serotonin, a neurotransmitter linked to emotions of wellbeing and relaxation.

Meal Plans to Lower Anxiety

Developing meal plans with the intention of lowering anxiety requires a well-rounded nutritional strategy that includes the items listed above. Here's how to organize meal plans for senior citizens who want to reduce their anxiety:

Breakfast: Have a well-balanced meal to start the day that includes fruits, whole grains, and a lean protein source. A healthy choice is a bowl of porridge with berries and a few almonds.

Lunch: Should emphasize a range of veggies, lean meats, and healthy fats. A fulfilling and calming meal can be fashioned out of a mixed green salad with grilled chicken and an olive oil and herb vinaigrette.

Dinner: Choose a well-balanced meal that consists of steamed vegetables, quinoa on the side, and a serving of fatty fish, such as salmon. Complex carbs, magnesium, and omega-3 fatty acids are provided by this combination.

Snacks: Select foods that are high in fiber, protein, and good fats. A tiny portion of Greek yogurt sweetened with honey and a small handful of mixed nuts will help keep blood sugar levels steady and lessen anxiety.

A senior's diet can benefit from including certain foods and meal plans since they can reduce anxiety and enhance mental health, which can lead to relaxation and general well-being.

CHAPTER 7:

MAINTAINING SOCIAL CONNECTIONS THROUGH FOOD

The Social Aspect of Dining

There is no denying the social aspect of dining when it comes to seniors' pursuit of optimal mental health and well-being. A person's mental health can be greatly enhanced by dining communally and sharing meals with close friends and family. This chapter examines the value of dining socially and how it might improve seniors' quality of life in general.

Cooking and Eating Advice for Those You Love

Family Get-Togethers: Plan frequent family get-togethers for meals so that generations can connect, exchange tales, and make enduring memories. These events can give people a feeling of purpose and belonging.

Cooking Together: Invite your loved ones to help you prepare meals. Cooking together improves social ties and creates a sense of accomplishment.

Potluck Dinners: Organizing potluck meals is a great way to get people to share their favorite dishes. This facilitates a wide variety of nutrient-dense foods and lessens the host's workload.

Themed Dinners: Investigate ethnic food nights or themed meals. These culinary explorations can be instructive as well as enjoyable, igniting interest and provoking discussions.

Picnics & Outside Dining: Eat outside whenever you can. It can be wonderful to dine outside and enjoy a change of scenery and fresh air.

Community Resources and Events

Senior Centers: Senior centers can serve as a focal point for senior socialization and engagement, offering meal programs, support services, and social activities.

Volunteer Opportunities: Seniors can gain a sense of purpose and make connections with others by volunteering at local food banks or events.

Culinary workshops: Seniors who are interested in meeting new people and learning new skills might take advantage of the culinary workshops that certain communities offer.

Dining Clubs: Meeting others who have similar interests and discovering new foods can be accomplished by joining a dining club or senior supper club.

Activities related to the Arts and Culture: Look into local activities related to the Arts and Culture that can include food, including cooking classes or food festivals. These gatherings can enhance culture while also being entertaining.

Seniors can improve their mental health by sharing meaningful experiences and meaningful connections with others by stressing the social side of meals and offering helpful cooking and dining with loved one's ideas.

Seniors can also take advantage of community programs and events to stay involved, active, and socially connected—all crucial components of living a long and happy life as they age.

"Mindful Eating, Mindful Living."

CHAPTER 8:

HEALTHY AGING AND LIFELONG MENTAL WELLNESS

Staying Active and Engaged in Later Life

Maintaining an active and involved lifestyle in later years is essential to senior mental health. The significance of sustaining social and physical exercise to support cognitive well-being is covered in this chapter. It offers helpful advice and insights on how seniors can fit an active lifestyle into their everyday schedule. This chapter covers the following subjects:

The advantages of physical activity: Talking about how regular exercise can improve mental health in general, elevate mood, and lower the risk of cognitive decline.

Adapting physical activity to your needs: Providing a variety of exercises appropriate for varying degrees of mobility and fitness, with a focus on the significance of discovering activities that senior citizens find enjoyable.

Participating in social activities: Emphasizing the benefits to mental health that come from upholding social links through volunteer work, group activities, or hobby pursuits.

Overcoming common barriers: This section discusses typical impediments, such as physical restrictions, that prevent people from being active and involved in their older years and offers solutions.

"Cooking Away the Blues: Recipes for a Brighter Day."

CHAPTER 9:

MINDFULNESS AND MENTAL WELL-BEING

Being mindful is an effective strategy for preserving mental health, and it's especially important for elders. This chapter explores mindfulness practices and how they affect cognitive health. It provides advice on how to apply mindfulness in day-to-day activities, including subjects like:

Understanding mindfulness: Defining mindfulness and outlining its possible advantages for lowering stress, strengthening emotional control, and boosting focus.

Mindful Eating: Talking about the benefits of mindful eating, which include discussing how eating with intention, appreciating food, and enjoying the sensory experience of meals, can improve mental and emotional well-being.

Exercises promoting mindfulness: Offering seniors useful methods and activities to practice mindfulness on a regular basis, which will help them unwind and improve their mental clarity.

Resources for mindfulness: recommending to seniors who want to learn more about and practice mindfulness books, apps, and community initiatives.

"Spice Up Your Life, Boost Your Mood."

CONCLUSION

We've set out to investigate the deep relationship between diet and mental health in the prime of life within the pages of this Mental Health Cookbook for Seniors. As a nutritionist, I have personally experienced how food can change our bodies and thoughts. With this expertise and enthusiasm, I offer you this culinary guide, which has been especially designed to meet the special requirements of our elderly community.

We have explored the role that good diet plays in preserving mental health, reducing stress and anxiety, and fostering social well-being throughout this cookbook. Through investigation, we have found a variety of nutrients that strengthen the brain and promote emotional stability, such as antioxidants and omega-3 fatty acids.

These meal plans and recipes are tools for fostering mental resilience and happiness, not just lists of recipes to follow. You can take proactive measures to protect your mental health and enjoy the richness of your senior years by implementing these delicious and nourishing dishes into your daily life.

Additionally, this cookbook promotes older citizens to spend quality time with loved ones over meals. Making and eating meals together strengthens social ties and helps fend off feelings of loneliness and isolation. Recall that not only are we what we eat, but also how we eat, and that sharing meals with others may bring about an immense sense of pleasure and satisfaction.

I encourage you to have a positive and determined approach to your nutritional journey as you embrace the culinary wisdom found inside these pages. It's possible that your golden years will be the most satisfying of your life.

You may cultivate the extraordinary person that you are, enhance your mental and emotional well-being, and cherish life's special moments with the proper foods, thoughtful ingredient selections, and mindful cooking practices.

Let this Mental Health Cookbook for Seniors be your culinary confidant and trusted partner going forward. I hope it gives you the confidence to manage your mental well-being and enjoy the benefits of your knowledge and life experiences. Accept the transformational power of food and relish each mouthwatering morsel. Your mental health is valuable, and the best is still to come.